Praise for

LADYBUG YOGA

"We are delighted to have Ladybug Yoga as a part of our enrichment program. It is a fantastic program and our kids enjoy it immensely. The teachers are dynamic and they understand the needs of the children perfectly. The Ladybug Yoga classes are fun, creative, and our children are happy to participate!

"There is a reason that this program is termed 'enrichment.' Ladybug Yoga enriches the lives of all the children who participate in it. It is an extremely positive program and the children learn how to connect with themselves in a friendly, relaxed environment. This is learning, at its optimum.

"I would highly recommend Ladybug Yoga Classes!"

—*Mike Jacobs, Saint Andrew's School*

"Ladybug Yoga has now been in our school for over six years. Children at our school thrive and look forward to each and every class. This program is very creative, lots of fun, and, more important, it teaches children simple tools to use at home and in school which help them with self-confidence and concentration, among many other positive benefits. I highly recommend Ladybug Yoga to schools and to parents. The results are astounding!"

—*Nancy Goldstein, Early Childhood Center Director,*
B'nai Torah Congregation

"For the past year, my three-year-old daughter has been taking Ladybug Yoga classes as a weekly after-school enrichment activity. She looks forward to 'yoga day' each week, and she is all smiles when she comes home. She enjoys demonstrating the various yoga positions she learns each week (downward-facing dog, tree pose, etc.), and telling us about the latest lessons with her friends in class.

"Over the past year, my daughter's balance and agility have improved dramatically. I attribute it in no small part to the Ladybug Yoga classes, which have given her age-appropriate methods to focus on her body and coordination. I appreciate that Ladybug Yoga also teaches her mindfulness and relaxation techniques, which carry over from class into her everyday routine.

"Ladybug Yoga provides a safe, fun, and enriching experience for my daughter, and the lessons will grow with her as she matures. I look forward to having her continue Ladybug Yoga classes in the future."

—*Nicole K., South Florida*

"I'm so grateful to Ladybug Yoga. After my daughter started taking classes, she really learned how to calm herself with the breathing techniques she learned. Whether it was to calm herself during a tantrum or when she felt anxious, she now does her breathing techniques or takes herself on a 'relaxation journey' as she does in class. It is so inspiring to see. I myself do yoga and wish I could've started at her young age. Such useful tools to deal with lifelong situations! Not only that, but her balance has increased, as well as her flexibility. She also dances and plays tennis, and I can't say enough good things about how these yoga classes have helped to improve her body condition and excel in her other activities. My daughter is much happier, which makes me one happy mommy! Thanks again, Ladybug Yoga!"

—*Stacy J., South Florida*

LADYBUG
YOGA

IN-CLASSROOM TEACHER TOOLS & TECHNIQUES GUIDE

SANDY GOLOGURSKY

Founder, Ladybug Yoga LLC

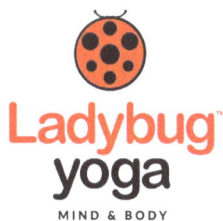

Ladybug
yoga
MIND & BODY

DISCLAIMER: The information provided in this book is intended for teachers to use in the classroom for short intervals throughout the school day. All forms of physical activity and exercise carry with them a risk of injury, and not all yoga practices and poses are suitable for everyone. Teachers must use their judgment and discretion during each class, with safety being paramount.

The author, Ladybug Yoga LLC, and its affiliates assume no responsibility or liability for any injuries or losses that might result from practicing yoga or engaging in any of the activities contained within this book. Should the reader have any questions concerning the appropriateness of any exercise or activity described, the author and Ladybug Yoga strongly suggest consulting a certified yoga instructor.

Published by
Ladybug Yoga LLC
Boca Raton, FL
www.theLadybugYoga.com
E-mail: Sandy@theladybugyoga.com
Facebook/LadybugYoga
Instagram/LadybugYoga

ISBN: 978-0-69298-241-9

Production by The Book Couple • www.thebookcouple.com

Contents

About Ladybug Yoga

LADYBUG YOGA is a unique children's yoga program that has been taught in yoga studios, preschools, private schools, charter schools, private classes, and summer camps throughout South Florida since 2009. We have witnessed that teaching these amazing tools to young children will build a positive foundation for their whole life. This program is designed for children ages 3 and up and utilizes practical tools that have no basis in any particular religious faith.

Yoga helps children develop important skills in a fun, non-competitive environment. Even at a young age, children often feel pressure at school academically and socially, plus the added stress of competitive organized sports makes it easy for boys and girls to become overly self-critical and lose confidence in themselves as they grow and change.

Our goal is to nurture a child's inner strength and self-acceptance while encouraging and challenging them to develop the following attributes:

- Strength
- Coordination
- Flexibility
- Concentration
- Sense of Calm

- Balance
- Body Awareness
- Better Focus
- Self-confidence

Incorporating Ladybug Yoga into the Classroom

With classroom schedules so full of daily activities, it would be challenging to add a full yoga class into the school day . . . but that's okay! Practicing yoga for even a few minutes each day is highly beneficial for both children and teachers.

When incorporating the Ladybug Yoga tools and techniques into your classroom, allow the children to be creative with their body movements. Never put them down or be critical if they are doing a pose incorrectly. Encourage the children to be themselves and to "shine as bright" as they can! Explain to them the importance of these tools and remind them to incorporate the Ladybug Yoga techniques at home, too.

Suggestions for when to incorporate Ladybug Yoga into your school day:

Body Awareness Time

◆ Any time of day

Breathing Exercises

◆ First thing in the morning

◆ Before having to concentrate for a long period of time

◆ Before and/or after a test

◆ When there is too much tension in the classroom

◆ Before and/or after transitioning

Yoga Poses

◆ To release lots of energy

◆ To get the children's attention

◆ After a snack or before lunch

◆ During recess

◆ After having to focus for an extended period

Suggestions for when to incorporate Ladybug Yoga into your school day (continued):

Games

◆ To have fun

◆ During recess

◆ If the class needs to take a break from a scheduled routine

◆ During rainy-day activity

◆ To release energy

◆ To promote team building, group connection, and concentration

Ladybug Yoga Moment

◆ Any time of day

Positive Affirmations

◆ During morning routine

Relaxation

◆ To recharge children's energy

◆ After sports activities

◆ Following time on the playground

◆ After lunch

◆ Before and/or after a test

◆ When children have too much energy and can't seem to focus

CLASSROOM SET-UP

Depending on the available time and circumstances, teacher can implement any or all of the following suggestions:

◆ If there are windows, turn off lights, allowing only natural light to come in. If there are no windows, dim lights.

◆ Play Ladybug Yoga class music to create a relaxing atmosphere.

◆ Children can be seated crisscross in a circle on the carpet or in their chair (at their desk) with their feet flat on the floor.

◆ It is suggested that the Ladybug Yoga Poses be done on a carpet or rug, and that Ladybug Yoga Chair Poses be done in their chairs.

Ladybug Yoga Body Awareness Time

BODY AWARENESS

At times during the school day, children can become fidgety or restless. Becoming aware of their bodies quickly calms the children and brings them into the present moment. When the children become aware of their bodies and are able to relax, they can move on to the next activity with more focus and concentration. It only takes about 30 seconds.

Have the children sit either crisscross on the carpet or at their desk with feet flat on the floor and hands on knees. Teacher says "Close your eyes. I want you to wiggle your toes (pause). Wiggle your fingers (pause). Wiggle your nose (pause). Put a beautiful smile on your face (pause). Feel your breath in your body (pause). Take a big inhale through your nose, making a big balloon in your belly, then exhale through your nose, letting it go. (Repeat breath 2 more times.) Now slowly open your eyes."

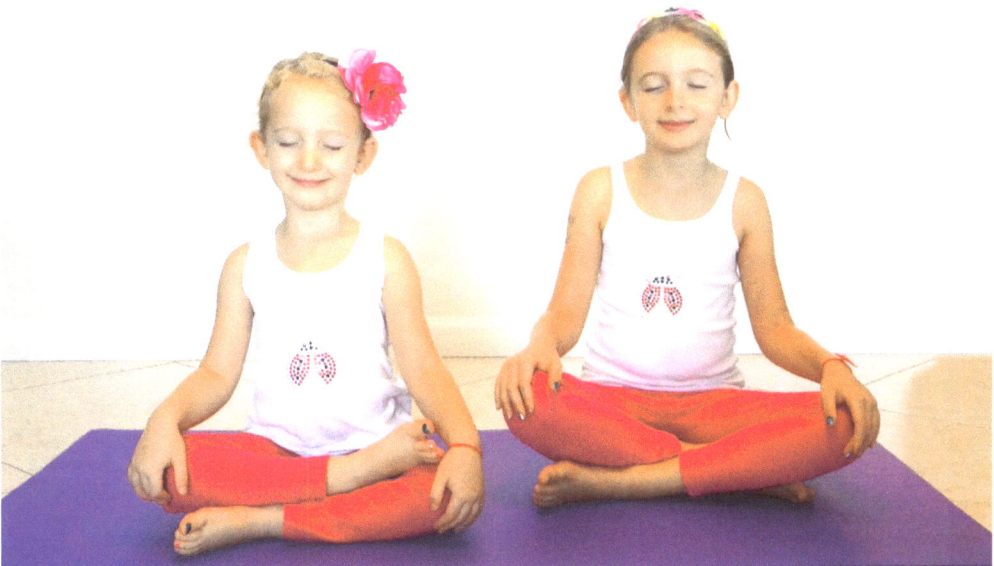

Ladybug Yoga Breathing Exercises

Breathing practice is very important for many reasons. To name a few: Breathing teaches children to turn inwardly and connect within themselves to experience, feel, gain control of, and understand their bodies. Breathing practice also trains their bodies to respond automatically to help calm themselves down at times when they are feeling stressed, anxious, or sad. Focused and correct forms of breathing are related to many positive benefits, including health, vitality, and happiness. By learning this important tool at a young age, children will have received the best gift possible for life!

Choose one breathing exercise per session. Time frame: 30 seconds to 5 minutes

Breathing exercises are done through the nose only, unless guided otherwise. Inhale through the nose, then exhale through the nose.

Inhale: Take a deep breath in through your nose.

Exhale: Release the breath out through your nose.

Hold: Hold the breath for the count.

CLAP BREATH

◆ Children sit crisscross on carpet or at their desk with feet on the floor.

◆ Teacher says, "Today we are doing the Clap Breath."

◆ Teacher instructs, "Place palms together to your heart center. Inhale, lift palms up to the sky above your head and clap. Exhale, bring palms back to your heart center." (Repeat 3 times.) "Inhale, palms up, hold your breath, and clap one, two. Exhale, bring palms back to your heart center." (Increase the number of claps. Repeat 4–8 times.)

SIGH BREATH

◆ Children sit crisscross on carpet or at their desk with feet on the floor. Hands on their knees.

◆ Teacher says, "Today we will do the Sigh Breath."

◆ Teacher instructs, "Big inhale through your nose and exhale out through your mouth, making a loud sighing noise." (Repeat 4–8 times.)

◆ Teacher explains that when the children breathe in, they breathe in happiness and other good feelings, and when they breathe out, they can let out any anger, sadness, or stress they may be feeling.

◆ Child can take turns suggesting something to inhale and something to exhale.

SUNSHINE BREATH

◆ Children sit crisscross on carpet or at their desk with feet on the floor. Arms by their sides and fingers spread.

◆ Teacher says, "Today we are going to do the Sunshine Breath."

◆ Teacher instructs, "Inhale through your nose, turn palms upward with fingers spread as you stretch your arms up and overhead with fingertips meeting, forming a round, bright sunshine with a big smile on your face. Then exhale, turn palms downward with fingers spread, bringing arms back down to your sides as we let our rays shine down." (Repeat 4 times.)

◆ Then, add a hold and increase holding the breath each time as arms are overhead "creating our sunshine." (Repeat 5 times.)

◆ For younger children, teacher can say, "Let's make a Sad sun. Angry sun. Silly sun. Tired sun, etc. . . ."

Ladybug Yoga Poses

The practice of yoga poses is very important, as the poses have many beneficial effects. Children develop strength, flexibility, and balance, while discovering that their minds and bodies are connected, which assists them in increasing their self-awareness, building their self-esteem, and helping them learn how to focus and concentrate.

The **Ladybug Yoga Poses** are designed for children of different ages. Each child has a different range of flexibility. It is important that the teacher is always conscious of each child's limitations and supports them at all levels while practicing the poses.

The symbol(s) next to each pose indicate its suggested age-appropriate level(s): **P** Preschool, **E+** Elementary and up.

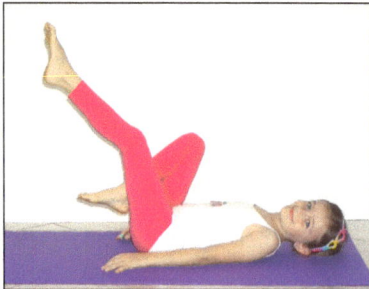

Bicycle Riding Pose (P, E+)—Lift legs up to the sky and start pedaling with legs forward, as if on a bicycle. Then pedal in reverse. (Older children can pedal in each direction for a count of 20–30.)

Teacher tells a story about the scenery they are passing while children are "riding their bikes."

Tiny Ball Pose (P, E+)—Hug knees into a tiny ball, and rock from side to side.

Teacher asks, "Who can get into the smallest ball?"

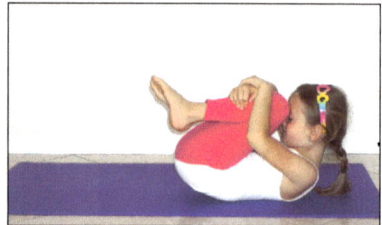

Ladybug Pose (P)—Bend knees and grab feet from the inside, knees drawing down to the floor and feet parallel to the sky.

Teacher says, "We are bugs on our backs. What type of bug are you today?"

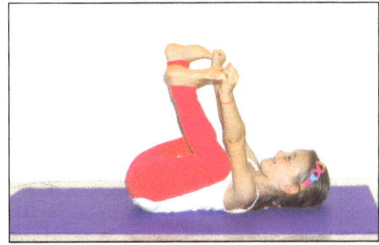

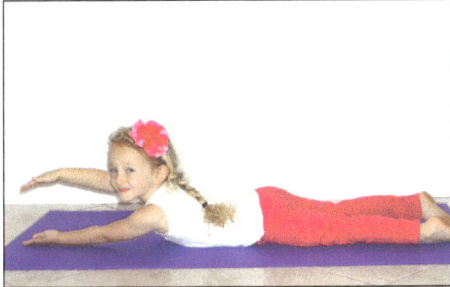

Crocodile Pose (P)—Lie on stomach, extend arms out in front, looking forward. Open and close arms.

Teacher and younger students say, "Chomp, chomp, chomp, chomp."

Boat Pose (P, E+)—Legs together, bend legs and bring feet off the floor, placing knees and feet parallel to the floor. Arms at the sides, moving as if rowing a boat. (Older children hold for a count of 10–20.)

Teacher and students sing "Row Your Boat."

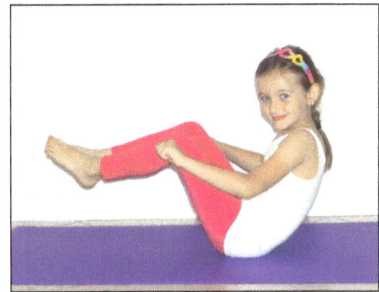

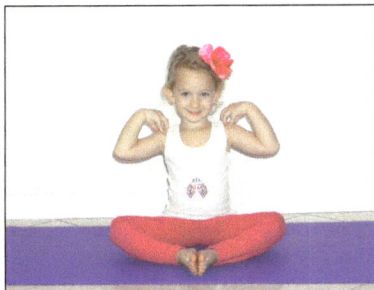

Butterfly Pose (P, E+)—Place soles of feet together, flapping knees, with hands on shoulders or on head as antennas. (Older children place hands on feet.)

Teacher asks, "Where are we traveling?" or "What color is your butterfly today?"

Crab Pose (Reverse Table) (P, E+)—Bend legs with feet flat on the floor. Place hands behind back flat on mat. Lift hips off the floor and raise one hand, opening and closing fingers as claws, lower the hand, then raise the other. (Older children lift one hand and opposite leg, finding balance. Hold for a count of 10, then switch.)

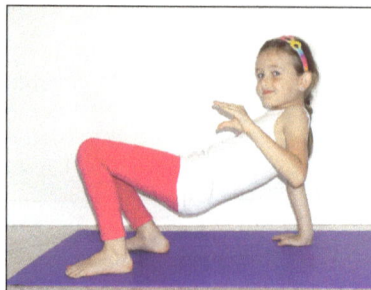

Teacher and students say, "Chomp, chomp." as they open and close their fingers.

Spider Fingers (P, E+)—Extend legs out in front. Show spider fingers (extended fingers as if spider legs) with hands in the air. Then, place fingers on thighs, walking spider fingers to toes (moving into a seated forward fold). Then walk spider fingers up and down and up. (Repeat a few times, going faster.) At the end, teacher says, "Now, let's hold our toes and count to ten."

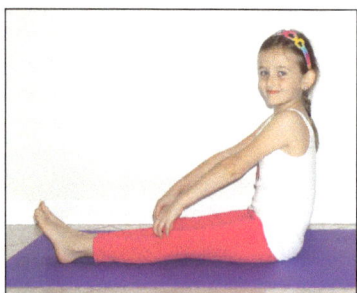

Baby Pose (P, E+)—Begin on knees with tops of feet flat on floor, then sit backside on heels, and bring head to the ground with arms along sides.

Teacher asks, "What do babies say?" Wah!

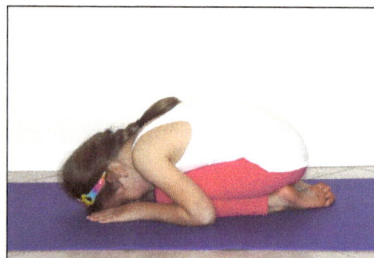

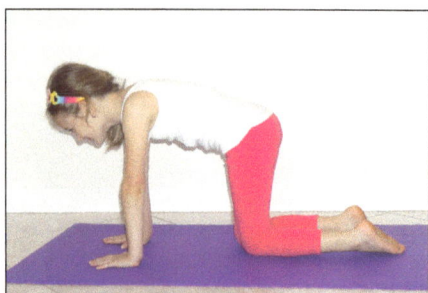

Table Pose (P, E+)—Place hands and knees on floor hip-width apart, neck and back straight with eyes gazing at the floor. Hold for a count of 5–10.

Teacher says, "Stay very still. Should someone eat breakfast, lunch, or dinner on us?"

Cat Pose (P, E+)—Begin in Table Pose, then round back, bringing chin to chest.

Teacher asks, "What do cats say?" Meowwwww!

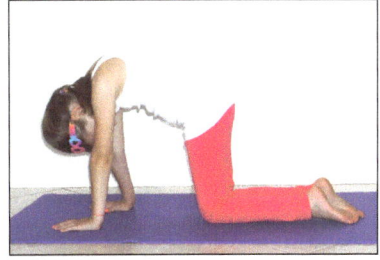

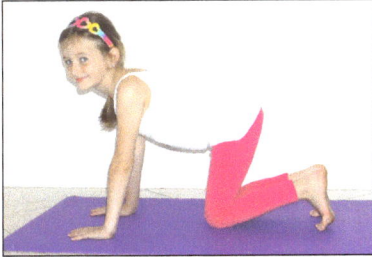

Cow Pose (P, E+)—Begin in Table Pose, then drop hips and shoulders back and look forward with chin slightly raised.

Teacher asks, "What do cows say?" Mooooo!

Dog Pose (P, E+)—Place hands under shoulders on the mat and lift hips to the sky with heels on the floor, eyes looking at knees. (Older children can lift one leg up, and then switch with the other leg. Then lift one leg and opposite hand, then switch.)

Teacher asks, "What does a dog say?" Woof! Woof!

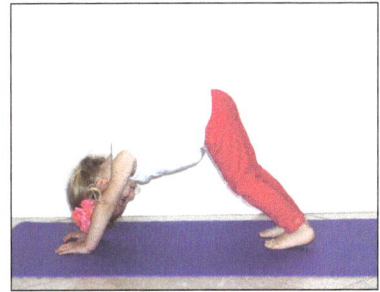

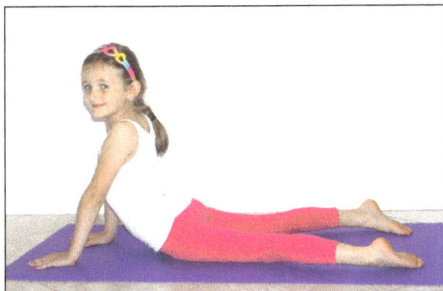

Snake Pose (P, E+)—Begin in Table Pose and bring hips forward onto the floor and lift chest, shoulders, and back.

Teacher asks, "What do snakes say?" Sssssssssss!

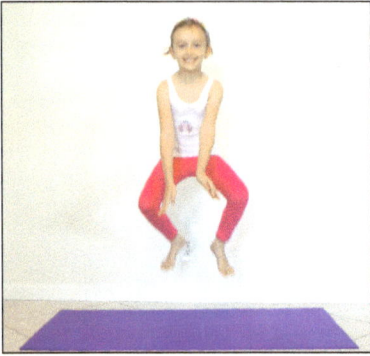

Frog Pose (P)—Feet on floor and place hands between feet. Hop as high as possible.

Teacher asks, "What does a frog say?" Ribbit, ribbit!

Teacher asks, "How high can you hop?" or "Who can hop up to the ceiling?"

Lion Pose (P)—On knees, lift torso up and place hands in front of chest with curled fingers.

Teacher asks, "What does a lion say?" Rrrrrrrrrrr!
Teacher jokes, "Oh, you scared me!"

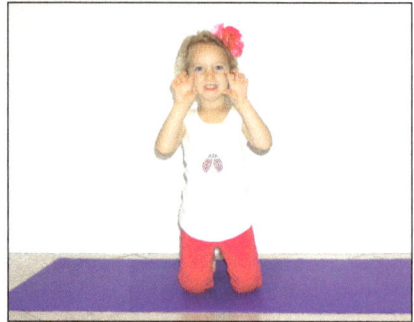

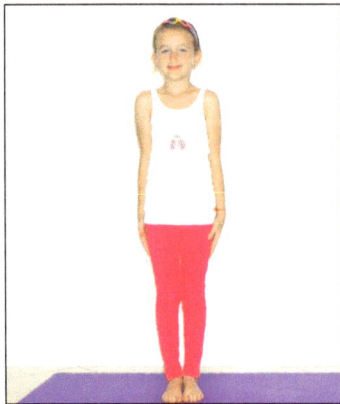

Mountain Pose (P, E+)—Stand with legs together and arms by sides and hold to be a tall mountain. Then take one hand and shield eyes, as if looking down at something.

Teacher says, "Stay very still and tall like a mountain."

Teacher asks, "What's at the bottom of your mountain?"

Forward Fold Touching Toes Pose (P, E+)— Standing in Mountain Pose, extend arms to the sky. Fold forward, touching toes, and hold for a count of 10. Roll all the way up.

Teacher says, "I'm touching my toes. Are you touching yours?"

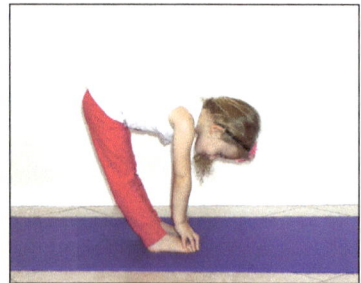

Dinosaur Pose (P)—Stand with feet wide apart and place hands on knees. Lift one knee at a time as high as possible while walking around the room.

Teacher asks, "How high can you lift your knees?" Teacher says, "Rrroarrr!"

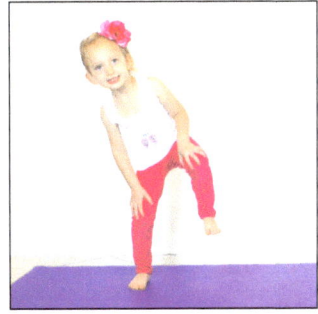

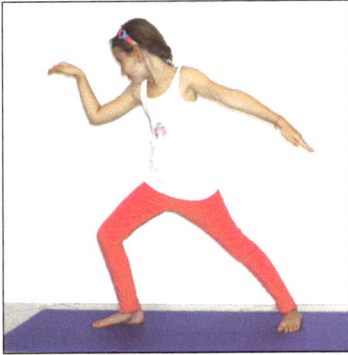

Elephant Pose (Warrior 2) (P, E+)—Open legs into a V and extend one knee over ankle and open arms parallel to floor using front arm as trunk, placed in front of chin, and back arm as tail, swaying trunk. Repeat on the other side. (Older children hold pose with straight arms parallel to the floor for a count of 20.)

Teacher says, "Heee, heee!"

Giraffe Pose (P)—Standing in Mountain Pose, extend arms straight up overhead with hands together, dropping fingers and locking thumbs. Walk with legs straight without bending knees. (Older children can walk on tippy-toes.)

Teacher asks, "What has a long neck and long legs?" or "What do giraffes eat?"

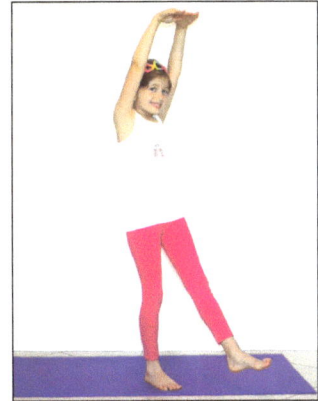

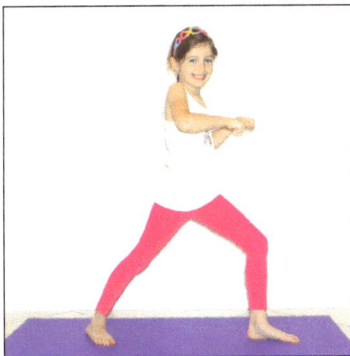

Horse Pose (Warrior 1) (P, E+)—Extend one leg forward, bending knee over ankle and place hands out in front as if holding onto a rope. Gallop around the room. Then switch legs. (Older children raise arms upward with palms facing and hold for a count of 20.)

Teacher says, "Let's climb onto our horsey." or "Giddy up, horsey, giddy up, horsey."

Kangaroo Pose (P)—Place legs, feet, and hands together and hop around.

Teacher says, "Hop, hop, hop! How high can you hop? How far can you hop?"

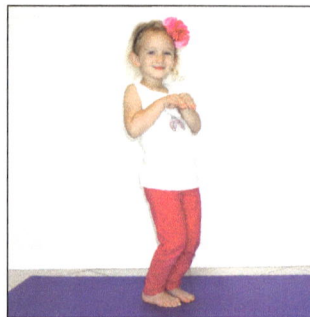

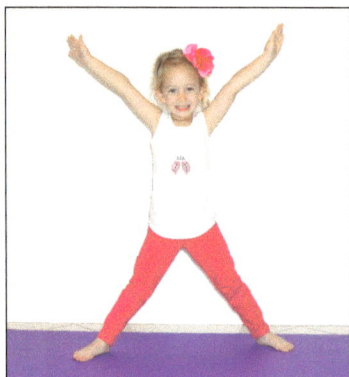

Shining Star Pose (P, E+)—Standing in Mountain Pose, jump arms and legs open to a shining star and smile. Hold. Then jump arms and legs together, back to Mountain Pose. Do this several times like jumping jacks.

Teacher says, "Smile like a shining star and hold." Teacher says, "Open and close and open and close." (Repeating and progressing faster each time.)

Airplane Pose (P, E+)—Standing in Mountain Pose, open arms parallel to the ground, creating airplane wings. Extend leg behind body parallel to the floor, finding balance, or fly around the room switching legs each step.

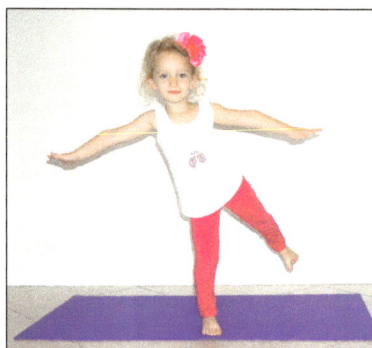

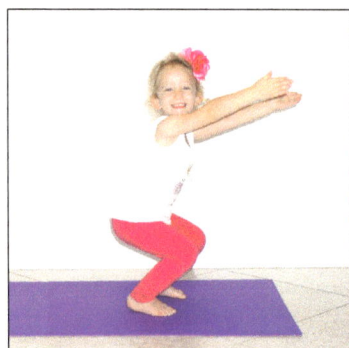

Chair Pose (P, E+)—Stand with feet hip-width apart and bend knees, dropping hips back and pretending to be sitting on a chair. Extend arms out front by ears.

Teacher asks, "Who's sitting in your chair?"

Flamingo Pose (P, E+)—Standing in Mountain Pose, lift knee up, bringing thigh parallel to floor. Bend arms, placing elbows to body and hands facing out as wings. Balance on one side, then hop and switch to the other leg. Balance on that side, then switch. (Older children lift knee and hold as high as they can for a count of 10–20.)

Teacher says, "Hop, hop, hop." Teacher asks, "What color is a flamingo?"

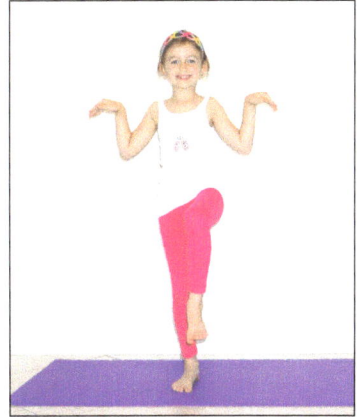

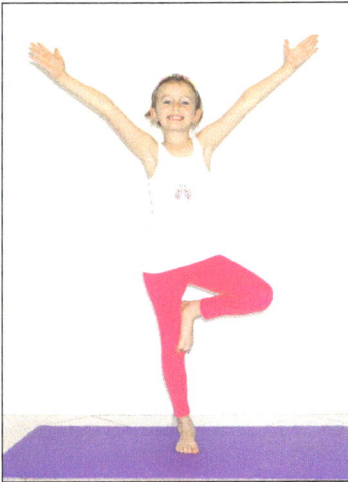

Tree Pose (P, E+)—Lift one foot up and place on thigh and place palms together to heart center. When balanced, extend arms up to create branches on a tree. Repeat on the other side and wave branches from side to side.

Teacher says, "Pick a spot to stare at and find your balance." Or "It's a windy day and our branches are swaying."

Triangle Pose (P, E+)—Open legs into a V shape and drop one arm, holding onto thigh, knee, or shin, extending other arm up to the sky while looking up. Repeat on the other side.

Teacher says, "Triangle."

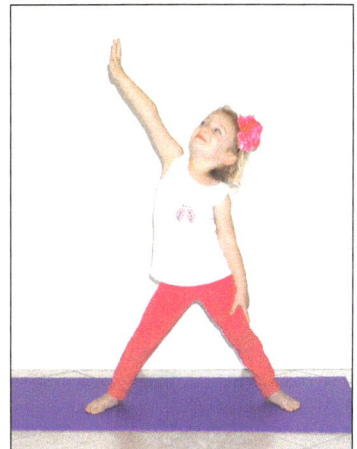

Ladybug Yoga Chair Poses

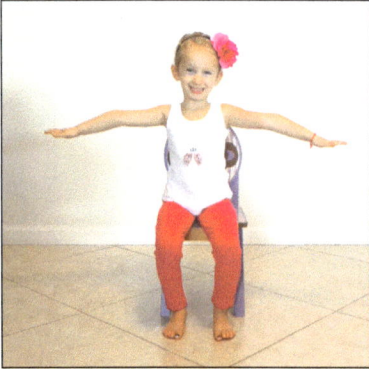

Airplane Arms Chair Pose (P, E+)—Open arms parallel to the ground, creating airplane wings. Sway side to side. (Older children can hold for a count of 10–30.)

Teacher says, "It's windy outside so sway your airplane wings." Teacher asks, "Where are you flying to?"

Dog Chair Pose (P, E+)—Stand facing chair. Place hands on seat of chair, moving feet slightly back. Hips up to the sky. Head in between arms and eyes looking at knees. (Older children can hold for a count of 10–20.)

Teacher asks, "What does a dog say?" Woof! Woof! "What color dog are you today?"

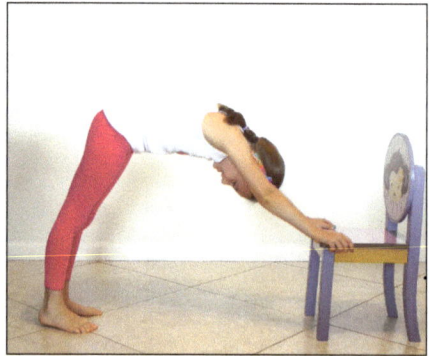

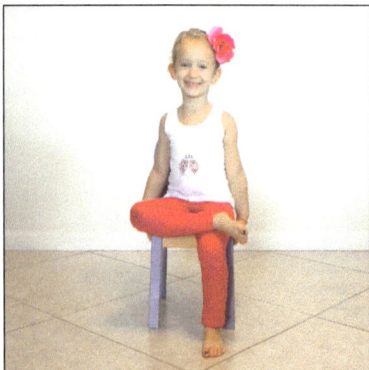

Half Lotus Chair Pose (P, E+)—Both feet flat on the floor. Bring right ankle to rest on left thigh. Keep knee in line with ankle as much as possible. Repeat on other side. Hold for a count of 5–10 on each side. (Older children can hold for a count of 10–20 on each side.)

Teacher asks, "What type of flower are you today?" or "What color flower are you?"

Side Stretch Chair Pose (P, E+)—Hang both arms down by sides. Extend right arm into the sky. Bend hip and reach fingers to opposite side. Repeat on other side.

Teacher says, "Ahhh, that feels so nice. What a great stretch!"

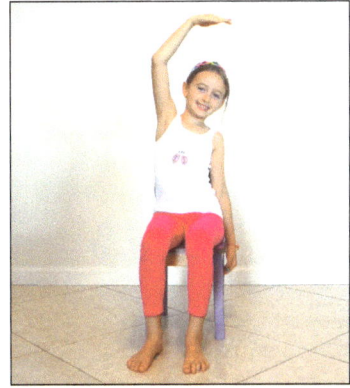

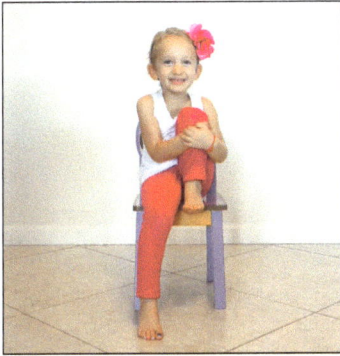

Hug Knee Chair Pose (P, E+)—Both feet flat on the floor. Lift right leg up, bring bent knee to chest and hug. Repeat on other side. (Older children can hold for a count of 10–20.)

Teacher says, "Give your knee a big hug!"

Seated Cat & Cow Chair Pose (P, E+)—Hands on knees. Lean forward, lengthen spine, and roll shoulders down and back, chin up (Cow Pose). Lean back, round spine, bring shoulders forward and drop chin to chest. (Cat Pose). Repeat a few times; more for older children.

Teacher asks, "What does a cat say?" Meowww! "What does a Cow say?" Mooo!

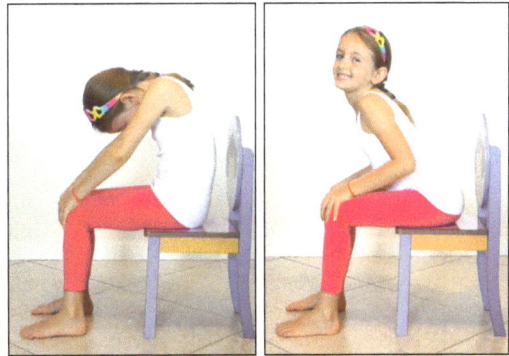

Touch Your Toes Chair Pose (P, E+)—Separate legs with feet flat on the floor. Stretch both arms up to sky. Fold forward and touch your toes. Hold for count of 5–10. (Older children can hold for a count of 10–20. Roll body all the way back up to seated.

Teacher says, "I'm touching my toes. Are you touching yours?"

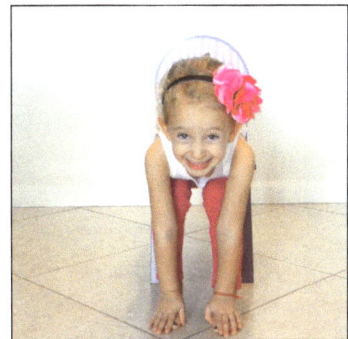

Tree Chair Pose (P, E+)—Stand next to chair with legs together and hands on hips with right side of body closer to chair. Hold chair with right hand. Lift left leg up and place foot on inside of thigh. Extend left arm up to sky. Hold for count of 5–10. (Older children can hold for a count of 10–20.) Repeat on other side.

Teacher says, "Pick a spot to stare at and find your balance."

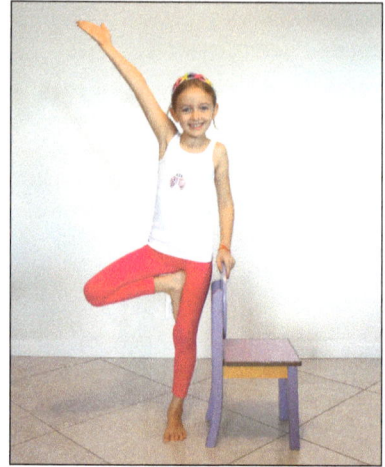

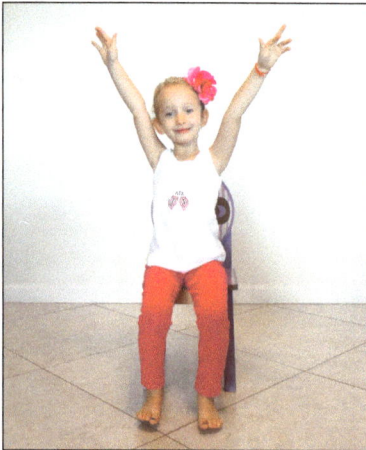

Twinkle Star Chair Pose (P, E+)—Extend both arms into the sky and twinkle fingers. (Older children can hold for a count of 10–30.)

Teacher says, "Twinkle your fingers!" Teacher and children sing "Twinkle, Twinkle, Little Star."

Washing Machine Chair Pose (P, E+)—Hands on shoulders. Twist side to side. Go faster and slower. (Older children can do more repetitions.)

Teacher says, "Twist from side to side washing your clothes! Go faster, faster, as fast as you can. Go slower, slower, as slow as you can."

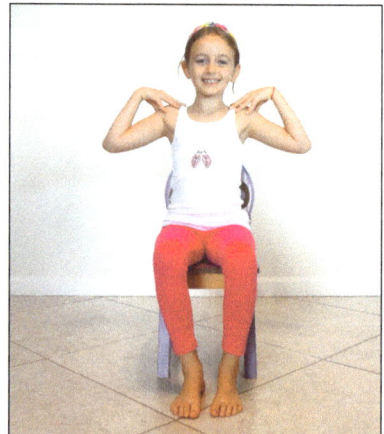

Ladybug Yoga Games

Each **Ladybug Yoga Game** incorporates various yoga poses found in this manual. Games are a time to have fun and interact with one another while receiving all the beneficial effects of the yoga poses. When deciding together which games to play during class, it is best to offer a variety of games as time permits. Games with an asterisk (*) next to the title indicate Ladybuy Yoga Essentials that can be purchased at www.theLadybugYoga.com.

DO THAT POSE GAME (P, E+)

Teacher names a yoga pose without demonstrating and children get into that pose. Any child who does not do the correct pose sits down. Play continues until only one child is left standing. That child receives a round of applause from all the children.

CONNECTED PARTNER POSES GAME (P, E+)

Teacher divides the children into partners. Teacher names a pose and partners do the pose, forming a "connected" yoga pose (attaching limbs in a creative manner).

HOLDING YOGA POSE GAME (P, E+)

Teacher chooses an appropriately challenging yoga pose. All children get into that pose and hold it for as long as they can. The last child holding the pose gets a round of applause from teacher and children. Teacher says, "Well done!" If a few children are still holding the pose and it has been a while, everyone counts to 10 and the children can come out of the pose. Teacher then chooses the next yoga pose.

LADYBUG YOGA LADYBUGS GAME* (P, E+)

Teacher hides the ladybugs around the room either before class or while children aren't looking. When all the ladybugs have been hidden, children walk around the room in various traveling animal poses. Teacher tells a story to lead the animals around the jungle, and then, when they get very hungry for dinner, they need to search for the ladybugs as their food. Teacher says, "Time for dinner!" and children start searching for the hidden ladybugs and pretending to eat them. Each child finds one ladybug. All ladybugs are then returned to the teacher.

LADYBUG YOGA WHAT'S IN THE BOX? GAME* (P, E+)

Teacher shows the children the special Ladybug Yoga box and says, "What's in the box? What's in the box?" Teacher places the box in the center of the circle. Going around the circle, each child picks a card out of the box. If the child can read, they read the card, and the class follows the request on the card. If the child cannot read yet, teacher reads the request. A couple of sample requests are:

◆ *Elephant Pose—Create your own elephant pose.*

◆ *Kangaroo Pose—How far can you hop?*

WASHING OUR CLOTHES GAME (P)

Children sit in a circle. Teacher asks, "Who has dirty clothes they need to wash?" Teacher goes around the circle, asking what each child needs to wash, and then everyone pretends to throw their clothes into the washing machine (the center of the circle).

Teacher demonstrates and explains, "Reach behind you and get the soap. Put some soap into the machine. Close the lid. Hands on your shoulders, turn the switch (your nose) to On!" Teacher and children say, "Beep," and twist from side to side saying, "Che che che che." Teacher says, "Make it go faster and faster . . . and stop! Let's open up the machine and look inside . . . OH! The clothes are clean, but they're wet. We need to dry them now, so let's put them into the dryer. . . . Close the door and put your hands on your knees. Turn the switch to On."

With hands on knees, teacher and children do full body circles from hips saying, "Gggggggrrrrrrrr." Teacher says, "Make it go faster and faster . . . and stop! Let's open up the dryer and look inside . . . OH yeah! They're dry." Teacher claps and says, "Good job! You all washed your own clothes today!"

YES I CAN GAME (P, E+)

Children stand and form a circle. Each child stands with legs together and open arms overhead, forming a Y with their body, representing the word "YES." Going around the circle, one at a time, each child takes a turn saying a positive affirmation beginning with "Yes, I can . . ." out loud, with energy and pride. For example: "Yes, I can dive into a swimming pool!" or "Yes, I can tie my shoes!" or "Yes, I can ride a bicycle!"

YOGA FREEZE (P, E+)

Teacher chooses a yoga pose and demonstrates to the class. Children dance in their spot. Then teacher claps hands and says, "FREEZE!" Children will freeze in the yoga pose the teacher demonstrated at the start of the round.

Teacher explains, "You are going to dance in place, and when I say FREEZE, you will freeze in the yoga pose I'm going to show you. The first pose is Tree Pose." (Demonstrate the pose each time.) "Dance in place, and FREEZE. Hold the pose. Good job! Next, you will freeze in a Snake Pose." (Again, demonstrate the pose.) "Dance in place, and FREEZE!" (Repeat, choosing a different pose each time.)

For part two of this game, teacher explains, "Next you will freeze in any yoga pose you choose. Think in your mind which pose you will freeze in, and let's dance in place . . . and FREEZE. If you are an animal, I want to hear your sounds. . . . Good job! Very creative!" (Repeat a few times.)

YOGA POSE MEMORY GAME (P)

Children and teacher sit in a circle. Teacher demonstrates a yoga pose, and the first child in the circle does that yoga pose and then adds another. The next child goes, doing both poses in order and adding a third. This continues around the circle, adding more and more poses until children and teacher feel challenged to remember.

YOGI SAYS (P, E+)

This is a variation of the game Simon Says. Instead of the command "Simon says," teacher uses the command "Yogi says." Children stand on the carpet, facing teacher. For example, teacher says and demonstrates, "Yogi says tree," or "Yogi says baby," and so on. Children get into the pose that "Yogi says."

If teacher says, "dog," but doesn't say, "Yogi says dog," children are not supposed to go into that pose. Teacher says, "Listen carefully and only do poses when Yogi says." If a child goes into pose without "Yogi says," they will sit down until only one child is left standing. (If there is time, children can take turns being Yogi.)

YOGI, YOGI, YOGA POSE (P)

This is a variation of the game Duck, Duck, Goose. Children sit in a circle. One child goes around gently tapping each head saying, "Yogi, Yogi, Yogi" until they choose a child and say a yoga pose instead. For example: "Yogi, Yogi, Yogi, Yogi, Elephant." The child chosen is in front of the tapping child as they do the yoga pose around the circle. The tapping child then sits in the open space, and the child chosen will now take a turn tapping. Each child can only be picked once so that no child gets excluded.

Take a Ladybug Yoga Moment

Below are **Ladybug Yoga Moments**. If you have 5–10 minutes and want to combine breathing with yoga poses, here are your go-to "moments." Pick one Moment to follow and repeat the steps as time permits. Combination poses are for children to switch back and forth to create a flow of energy in their bodies.

After completing the chosen Ladybug Yoga Moment, finish with Ladybug Yoga Body Awareness Time (see page 5).

#1 Moment

◆ 5 Sigh Breaths.

◆ 5 Cat & Cow combination poses.

◆ Boat Pose. Hold for a count of 10.

◆ Tree Pose. Find balance on each side.

#2 Moment

◆ 5 Sunshine Breaths.

◆ 5 Baby & Snake combination poses.

◆ Crab Pose. Hold for a count of 10.

◆ Airplane Pose. Find balance on each side.

#3 Moment

◆ 5 Clap Breaths.

◆ 5 Dog & Butterfly combination poses.

◆ Elephant Pose. Hold for a count of 10.

◆ Flamingo Pose. Find balance on each side.

#4 Moment

◆ 5 Sigh Breaths.

◆ 5 Crocodile & Frog combination poses.

◆ Shining Star Pose. Hold for a count of 10.

◆ Tree Pose. Find balance on each side.

#5 Moment

- 5 Sunshine Breaths.

- 5 Forward Fold Touching Toes & Chair combination poses.

- Table Pose. Hold for a count of 10.

- Flamingo Pose. Find balance on each side.

#6 Moment

- 5 Clap Breaths.

- 5 Kangaroo & Dinosaur combination poses.

- Bicycle Riding Pose. Pedal for a count of 10.

- Tree Pose. Find balance on each side.

#7 Moment

- 5 Sigh Breaths.

- 5 Triangle & Tiny Ball combination poses.

- Mountain Pose. Hold for a count of 10.

- Airplane Pose. Find balance on each side.

#8 Moment

- 5 Sunshine Breaths.

- 5 Shining Star & Spider Fingers combination poses.

- Lion Pose. Hold for a count of 10.

- Tree Pose. Find balance on each side.

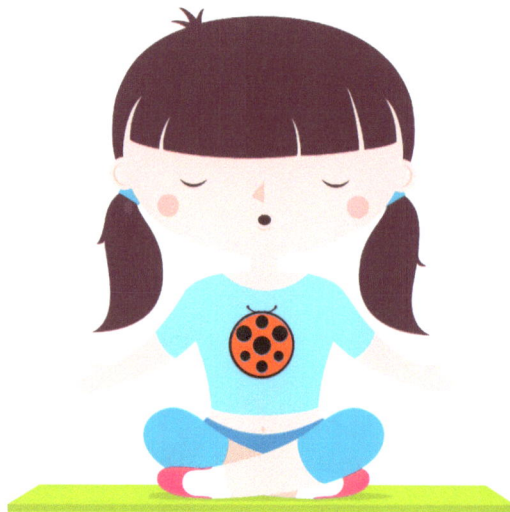

Ladybug Yoga Positive Affirmations

Positive affirmations are very important in our daily lives. Our thoughts create our feelings, which then ripple into our reality. It is important for children to learn this skill in order to focus on the beauty and positivity around and within themselves, as life will always offer challenges. Teaching children this tool will strengthen self-esteem and further the practice of mind over matter, which will assist them in overcoming obstacles they may encounter throughout their lives.

Teacher chooses one Ladybug Yoga Positive Affirmation for the school week or has each child choose an affirmation of their own. Children will share this affirmation with their classmates each day during the morning routine.

In the game section, you will find the "YES I Can . . . Game." This is a fun game that helps to build self-esteem.

Here are some affirmations to share with the class. Teacher can also have students suggest their own affirmations.

◆ I Am Happy   ◆ I Am Brave   ◆ I Am Sharing

◆ I Am Strong   ◆ I Believe in Myself   ◆ I Am Peaceful

◆ I Am Funny   ◆ I Am Beautiful   ◆ I Trust in Myself

◆ I Am Loved   ◆ I Am Caring   ◆ I Can Do It!

◆ I Am Smart

Ladybug Yoga Guided Relaxations

Relaxation is a an essential skill for children to learn. During this time, children can fully surrender their bodies, as they are able to slow down and be in the present moment. By taking this time, they are allowing their bodies to balance and rejuvenate while calming their minds. Teaching children these tools for how to stay in a place of calmness can benefit them greatly in their daily lives.

Choose one Ladybug Yoga Guided Relaxation to incorporate into each session. Time frame: 30 seconds to 5 minutes

CLOUD JOURNEY RELAXATION

Children sit at their desk or lie on the carpet in their own space. Teacher puts on Ladybug Yoga Class Music* and turns the lights off (if there are no windows in the classroom, then dim lights as much as possible). Teacher asks children to close their eyes.

Teacher says, "I want you to use your imagination, your mind, and I want you to climb up on a big, puffy cloud. Get comfy on this big, puffy cloud. Once you are as comfy as can be, imagine that the cloud takes off into the sky. One, two, three. You are flying through the clouds. The wind is brushing through your hair. You are traveling to a far-away place. You feel the sun shining on your face. You are so happy right now. You have no worries right now. You are having so much fun flying on this big, puffy cloud. Put a beautiful smile on your face. Relax your body and enjoy this special, special journey you are on." (Teacher is silent for a few moments.)

Teacher then says, "Now we need to travel back to the classroom, so let your cloud travel you back. Three, two, one. You have landed back in class. Take a deep breath as you stretch your arms overhead. Now slowly open your eyes."

WHOLE BODY RELAXATION

Children sit at their desk or lie on the carpet in their own space. Teacher puts on Ladybug Yoga Class Music* and turns the lights off (if there are no windows in the classroom, then dim lights as much as possible). Teacher asks children to close their eyes.

Pausing for a moment between statements, teacher says, "We are going to calm your body. So relax your toes. Relax your feet. Relax your ankles. Relax your legs. Relax your knees. Relax your hips. Relax your back. Relax your stomach. Relax your shoulders. Relax your arms. Relax your elbows. Relax your hands. Relax your fingers. Relax your neck. Relax your throat. Relax your head. Relax your eyes. Relax your ears. Relax your cheeks. Relax your nose. Relax your chin. Relax your mouth. Relax your teeth. Relax your tongue. Relax your hair. Relax your spine. Relax your whole body. Be calm. Relax your mind. Listen to the music and stay calm. You are all doing a wonderful job! Put a beautiful smile on your face. Just relax. Just relax." (Teacher is silent for a few moments, then repeats, "Just relax. Just relax." Again, teacher is silent for a few moments.)

Teacher then says, "Slowly, I want you to wiggle your toes, wiggle your fingers, open your eyes, and stay calm. Stretch your arms overhead and get a nice stretch."

---

*Ladybug Yoga Class Music is available at www.theLadybugYoga.com

A Note from Sandy
Founder of Ladybug Yoga

The **Ladybug Yoga** curriculum was created as an extension of my heart and soul. When I look back over my life, I see two main themes developing: the first is my role as a natural yogi, and the second is my role as a compassionate teacher.

As a young child who was raised by a health-conscious mother, I was afforded the opportunity to sit in on many yoga classes. I remember enjoying the yoga classes, even at an early age, and feeling right at home in the yoga studio. Yoga became a passion for me early on.

My other passion was being a role model and caretaker for young kids. I spent many summers working as a camp counselor, and after graduating high school, I became an Early Childhood Educator and taught for a few years. I adored working with children in this realm, but felt that an important piece of teaching was missing for me. I knew deep inside that I needed to expand on my formal training as an ECE and learn more about the ancient practice of yoga that I had been exposed to.

In 2004, after leaving Canada and moving to Florida to join my family, I found a highly revered yoga teacher training program: Nosara Yoga Institute in Costa Rica. Upon completing my RYT-200 (Registered Yoga Teacher) certification, I returned home and completed my RCYT (Registered Children's Yoga Teacher) training. I began teaching both adults and children in local yoga studios. I was extremely fortunate to have had the support and ongoing teachings of an amazing mentor who took me under her wing and guided me to flourish.

In 2009—when my first daughter, Maya, was born—it all came together for me, and I was inspired to combine my Early Childhood Education with my yoga training. That was exactly the instant—the "aha!" moment—in which **Ladybug Yoga** was created! I set out to create an original children's yoga program that teaches the most incredible, practical tools that kids can use in their everyday lives.

Other teachers soon joined me for the **Ladybug Yoga** adventure. We have been teaching children three years and older in schools and facilities throughout South Florida. As a result, the children, their parents, and the schools have witnessed firsthand how kids can benefit from such a curriculum.

I've received an abundance of interest from yoga instructors, teachers, parents, schools, and therapists to learn our program so that they can implement its lessons and tools in their own work with children, as well as with their own children at home. This interest led to my second "aha!" moment: I realized that it was time to create this program, which I now have the pleasure of presenting to you. This labor of love has evolved over the years into the Ladybug Yoga curriculum, and I invite you to share it with the children in your life.

—Sandy Gologursky, ECE, E-RYT 200, RCYT, YACEP

About the Author

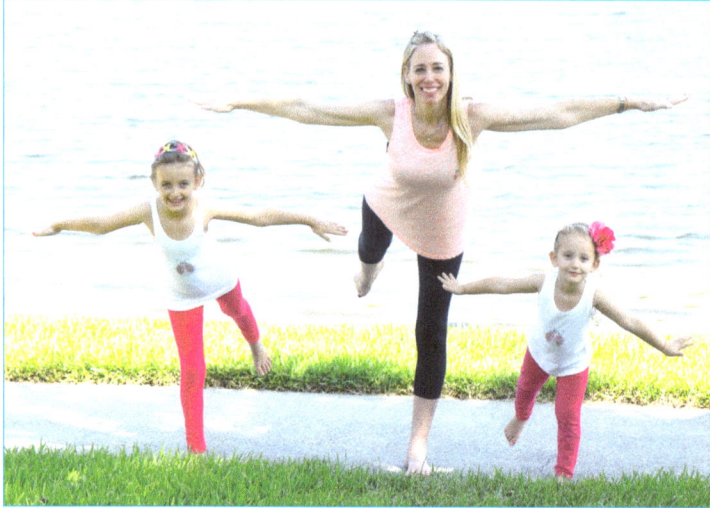

Sandy Gologursky, ECE, E-RYT 200, RCYT, YACEP, is the creator of the Ladybug Yoga system. She is a passionate advocate for Yoga practice for children. She believes that providing appropriate tools to parents and teachers will help them to make a positive difference in the lives of children as they grow and develop.

Contact Sandy at contact@LadybugYoga.com
or visit www.theLadybugYoga.com

Continue the Learning

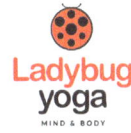

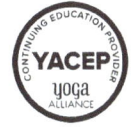

Ladybug Yoga is here to provide you with various guides and workshops for you to continue learning, which will truly assist you in your journey of sharing these amazing tools and techniques with children. Here are our recommended workshops & guides to further your education. They are all available at www.theLadybugYoga.com.

LADYBUG YOGA CHILDREN'S TEACHER TRAINING (IN-PERSON / ONLINE)*

Ladybug Yoga Children's Teacher Training is a dynamic, interactive, and fun training program geared toward anyone seeking to work with or currently working with children.

Expand your business, grow your clientele, and add a new branch of teaching by learning our practical, useful tools and techniques that will enable you to share the benefits of yoga with children to help them in their everyday lives!

After completion of this training, you will feel confident and excited to share these incredible new skills with children!

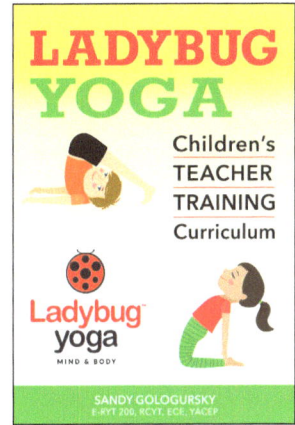

LADYBUG YOGA AT-HOME PARENT TOOLS & TECHNIQUES GUIDE

Ladybug Yoga At-Home Parent Tools & Techniques is a fun and interactive go-to guide that teaches parents how to share these useful tools and techniques with their children.

We understand that our children's schedules–being so overwhelmed with homework and after-school programs, plus all their regular responsibilities–doesn't give them much time to stop and have a full yoga class during the day . . . but that's okay! Practicing yoga for even a few minutes each day is highly beneficial for both children and their parents.

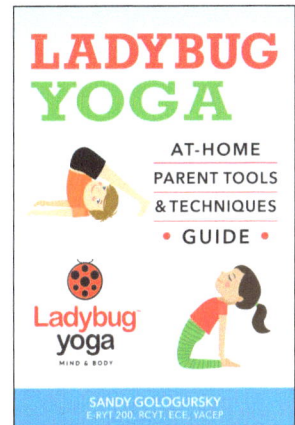

LADYBUG YOGA 8-WEEK SESSION PROGRAM PLAN

After completing the Ladybug Yoga Children's Teacher Training, it is now time for you to go out and positively impact the lives of children throughout the world!

Since it can be overwhelming and stressful at first to create your lesson plans, Ladybug Yoga created the **Ladybug Yoga 8-Week Session Program Plan** to make it easier on you from start to finish!

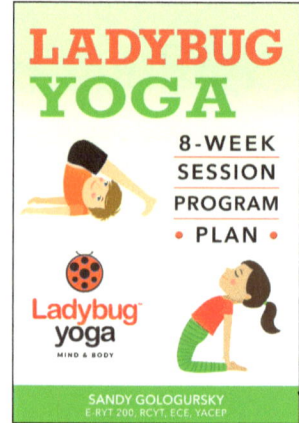

STEP-BY-STEP STARTUP GUIDE TO A CHILDREN'S YOGA BUSINESS

This is a very exciting time, as you are getting ready to embark on—and flourish in—your new venture! Your mind is exploding with amazing ideas, but you need assistance with the practical steps to take to get your business up and running—and have fun at the same time.

Let the **Step-by-Step Startup Guide to a Children's Yoga Business** show you how easy it can be to start your own thriving yoga business!

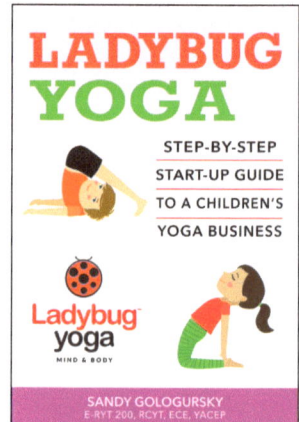

---

*Ladybug Yoga Children's Teacher Training is recognized as a Yoga Alliance Continuing Education Provider (YACEP). Registered Yoga Instructors can use this certification towards their Yoga Alliance Continuing Education (CE) hours. For more information on Ladybug Yoga certification, please contact Ladybug Yoga at contact@LadybugYoga.com or visit www.theLadybugYoga.com.

www.ingramcontent.com/pod-product-compliance
Lightning Source LLC
Chambersburg PA
CBHW060819270326
41930CB00002B/88